Air Fryer Quick & Easy Recipes

Collection of Side Dishes to Boost Your Air Fryer Meals

Franck McMillan

TABLE OF CONTENT

medical or professional advice. The content within this book has been derived from various sources. Please consult a licensed professional before attempting any techniques outlined in this book.

By reading this document, the reader agrees that under no circumstances is the author responsible for any losses, direct or indirect, which are incurred as a result of the use of information contained within this document, including, but not limited to, — errors, omissions, or inaccuracies.

Italian Pork Milanese

Preparation Time: 20 minutes

Cooking Time: 10 minutes

Servings: 46

Ingredients:

- 6 pork chops, center cut
- 2 eggs
- 2 tbsp. water
- cup panko bread crumbs seasoned with salt and black pepper
- 1/2 cup all-purpose flour
- Parmesan cheese, for serving (optional)
- tbsp. extra virgin olive oil
- For arugula salad:
- bag fresh arugula
- tbsp. freshly squeezed lemon juice
- 1 tsp. Dijon mustard
- 1/8 cup extra virgin olive oil
- Freshly ground black pepper and sea salt to taste

Directions:

1. Use a mallet or rolling pin to pound each pork chop into 1/4-inch cutlets.

2. Season well with salt and pepper then dip each cutlet in the flour. Shake off the excess.

3. Whisk the eggs with the water in a shallow bowl and dip the floured cutlets in the mixture then roll in the bread crumbs.

4. Do this for all the chops and set aside.

5. Set your air fryer toast oven at 380 degrees F.

6. Lightly brush the breaded pork chops with olive and arrange in one layer on your air fryer toast oven's basket. Cook for 3-5 minutes then flip the chops and cook for another 3-5 minutes or until golden and crisp.

7. Meanwhile, Directions: are the salad by combining the mustard, lemon juice, salt and pepper in a large bowl. Toss the arugula with the vinaigrette until evenly coated.

8. Serve the arugula salad and top with crisp cutlets and parmesan cheese (optional). Enjoy!

Nutrition: Calories: 417 kcal, Carbs: 23.8 g, Fat: 21.3

g, Protein: 20.1 g.

Air Roasted Jerk Pork

Preparation Time:10 minutes

Cooking Time: 1 hour 10 minutes

Servings: 10

Ingredients:

- 1800g pork shoulder
- tbsp. olive oil
- 1/4 cup Jamaican Jerk spice blend
- 1/2 cup beef broth
- Directions:
- Rub the roast with oil and dust with spice blend; set your air fryer toast oven to 400 degrees F and air roast on both sides for 4 minutes on each side in a large pan.
- Let rest for about 5 minutes before removing from oven.
- Shred and serve.

Nutrition: Calories: 298 kcal, Carbs: 7.4 g, Fat: 21.3 g, Protein: 19.6 g.

Apple and Carrot Stuffed Rotisserie Turkey

Preparation Time:30 minutes

Cooking Time: 3 hours

Servings: 12 to 14

<u>Ingredients:</u>

- (12-pound/5.4-kg) turkey, giblet removed, rinsed and pat dry
- For the Seasoning:
- ¼ cup lemon pepper
- tablespoons chopped fresh parsley
- 1 tablespoon celery salt
- cloves garlic, minced
- teaspoons ground black pepper
- 1 teaspoon sage
- For the Stuffing:
- 1 medium onion, cut into 8 equal parts
- 1 carrot, sliced
- 1 apple, cored and cut into 8 thick slices

Directions:

1. Mix together the seasoning in a small bowl. Rub over the surface and inside of the turkey.

2. Stuff the turkey with the onions, carrots, and apples. Using the rotisserie spit, push through the turkey and attach the rotisserie forks.

3. If desired, place aluminum foil onto the drip pan. (It makes for easier clean-up!)

4. Select the Roast function and preheat Maxx to 350 degrees Fahrenheit (180 degrees Celsius). Press ROTATE button and set Time to 3 hours.

5. Once preheated, place the turkey with rotisserie spit into the oven.

6. When cooking is complete, the internal temperature should read at least 180 degrees Fahrenheit (82 degrees Celsius). Remove the lamb leg using the rotisserie handle and, using hot pads or gloves, carefully remove the turkey from the spit.

7. Server hot.

Nutrition: Calories 274 Fat 12g Fiber 3g Protein 14g Carbohydrates 5g

Honey Glazed Rotisserie Ham

Preparation Time:20 minutes

Cooking Time: 3 hours

Servings: 6

Ingredients:

- (5-pound/2.3-kg) cooked boneless ham, pat dry
- For the Glaze:
- ½ cup honey
- teaspoons lemon juice
- 1 teaspoon ground cloves
- 1 teaspoon cinnamon
- ½ cup brown sugar

Directions

1. Using the rotisserie spit, push through the ham and attach the rotisserie forks.
2. If desired, place aluminum foil onto the drip pan. (It makes for easier clean-up!)
3. Select the Roast function and preheat Maxx to 250 degrees Fahrenheit (121 degrees Celsius). Press Rotate button and set Time to 3 hours.

4. Once preheated, place the ham with rotisserie spit into the oven.

5. Meanwhile, combine the Ingredients: for the glaze in a small bowl. Stir to mix well.

6. When the ham has reached 145 degrees Fahrenheit (63 degrees Celsius), brush the glaze mixture over all surfaces of the ham.

7. When cooking is complete, remove the ham using the rotisserie handle and, using hot pads or gloves, carefully remove the ham from the spit.

8. Let it rest for 10 minutes covered loosely with foil and then carve and serve.

Nutrition: Calories 473.0 Total Fat 17.1g Saturated Fat 9.3g Total Carbohydrate 53.8g Dietary Fiber 2.2g Sugars 12.7g Protein 23.0g

Bourbon Rotisserie Pork Shoulder

Preparation Time:30 minutes

Cooking Time: 4 hours 30 minutes

Servings: 6 to 8

Ingredients:

- (5-pound / 2.3-kg) boneless pork shoulder
- 1 tablespoon kosher salt
- For the Rub:
- teaspoons ground black peppercorns
- teaspoons ground mustard seed
- tablespoons light brown sugar
- 1 teaspoon onion powder
- 1 teaspoon garlic powder
- 1 teaspoon paprika
- For the Mop:
- 1 cup bourbon
- 1 small onion, granulated
- ¼ cup corn syrup
- ¼ cup ketchup
- tablespoons brown mustard
- ½ cup light brown sugar

Directions:

1. Combine the Ingredients: for the rub in a small bowl. Stir to mix well.

2. Season pork shoulder all over with rub, wrap in plastic, and place in refrigerator for 12 to 15 hours.

3. Remove roast from the fridge and let meat stand at room temperature for 30 to 45 minutes. Season with kosher salt.

4. Whisk Ingredients: for mop in a medium bowl. Set aside until ready to use.

5. Using the rotisserie spit, push through the pork should and attach the rotisserie forks.

6. If desired, place aluminum foil onto the drip pan. (It makes for easier clean-up!)

7. Select the Roast function and preheat Maxx to 450 degrees Fahrenheit (235 degrees Celsius). Press Rotate button and set Time to 30 minutes.

8. Once preheated, place the pork with rotisserie spit into the oven.

9. After 30 minutes, reduce the temperature to 250 degrees Fahrenheit (121 degrees Celsius) and roast for 4 more hours or until a meat thermometer inserted in the center

of the pork reads at least 145 degrees Fahrenheit (63 degrees Celsius).

10. After the first hour of cooking, apply mop over the pork for every 20 minutes.

11. When cooking is complete, remove the pork using the rotisserie handle and, using hot pads or gloves, carefully remove the pork tenderloin from the spit.

12. Let stand for 10 minutes before slicing and serving.

Nutrition: Calories 274.1 Total Fat 15.7g Saturated Fat 3.5g Total Carbohydrate 10.3g Dietary Fiber 1.1g Sugars 9.0g Protein 21.4g

Marinated Medium Rare Rotisserie Beef

Preparation Time:15 minutes

Cooking Time: 1 hour 40 minutes

Servings: 6 to 8

Ingredients:

- pounds (2.3 kg) eye round beef roast
- onions, sliced
- cups white wine
- cloves garlic, minced
- teaspoon chopped fresh rosemary
- 1 teaspoon celery seeds
- 1 teaspoon fresh thyme leaves
- ¾ cup olive oil
- 1 tablespoon coarse sea salt
- 1 tablespoon ground black pepper
- 1 teaspoon dried sage
- tablespoons unsalted butter

Directions:

1. Place beef roast and onions in a large resealable bag.

2. In a small bowl, combine the wine, garlic, rosemary, celery seeds, thyme leaves, oil, salt, pepper, and sage.

3. Pour the marinade mixture over the beef roast and seal the bag. Refrigerate the roast for up to one day.

4. Remove the beef roast from the marinade. Using the rotisserie spit, push through the beef roast and attach the rotisserie forks.

5. If desired, place aluminum foil onto the drip pan. (It makes for easier clean-up!)

6. Select the Roast function and preheat Maxx to 400 degrees Fahrenheit (205 degrees Celslus). Press Rotate button and set Timc to 1 hour 40 minutes.

7. Once preheated, place the lamb leg with rotisserie spit into the oven. Baste the beef roast with marinade for every 30 minutes.

8. When cooking is complete, remove the lamb leg using the rotisserie handle and, using hot pads or gloves, carefully remove the lamb leg from the spit.

9. Remove the roast to a platter and allow the roast to rest for 10 minutes.

10.   Slice thin and serve.

Nutrition: Calories 358.0 Total Fat 15.5g Saturated Fat 4.5g Total Carbohydrate 0.0g Dietary Fiber 0.0g Sugars 0.0g Protein 50.0g

Sriracha Honey Pork Tenderloin

Preparation Time: 20 minutes

Cooking Time: 25 minutes

Servings: 2 to 3

Ingredients:

- pound (454 g) pork tenderloin
- tablespoons Sriracha hot sauce
- tablespoons honey
- 1½ teaspoons kosher salt

Directions

1. Stir together the Sriracha hot sauce, honey and salt in a bowl. Rub the sauce all over the pork tenderloin.

2. Using the rotisserie spit, push through the pork tenderloin and attach the rotisserie forks.

3. If desired, place aluminum foil onto the drip pan. (It makes for easier clean-up!)

4. Select the Air Fry function and set the temperature to 350 degrees Fahrenheit (180 degrees Celsius). Press Rotate button and set Time to 20 minutes.

5. Place the pork tenderloin with rotisserie spit into the oven.

6. When cooking is complete, remove the pork tenderloin using the rotisserie handle and, using hot pads or gloves, carefully remove the chicken from the spit.

7. Let rest for 5 minutes and serve.

Nutrition: Calories 274.1 Total Fat 15.7g Saturated Fat 3.5g Total Carbohydrate 10.3g Dietary Fiber 1.1g Sugars 9.0g Protein 21.4g

Rotisserie Chicken with Lemon

Preparation Time:10 minutes

Cooking Time: 40 minutes

Servings: 6

Ingredients:

- (4 pounds / 1.8 kg) whole chicken
- teaspoons paprika
- 1½ teaspoons thyme
- 1 teaspoon onion powder
- 1 teaspoon garlic powder
- Salt and pepper, to taste
- ¼ cup butter, melted
- tablespoons olive oil
- 1 lemon, sliced
- sprigs rosemary

Directions

1. Remove the giblets from the chicken cavity and carefully loosen the skin starting at the neck.

2. In a bowl, mix together the paprika, thyme, onion powder, garlic powder, salt, and pepper. Set aside.

3. Rub the melted butter under the skin and pat the skin back into place.

4. Truss the chicken, ensuring the wings and legs are tied closely together and the cavity is closed up.

5. Drizzle the olive oil all over the chicken and rub it into the chicken.

6. Rub the spice mixture onto the chicken's skin.

7. Place the lemon slices and sprigs of rosemary into the cavity.

8. Using the rotisserie spit, push through the chicken and attach the rotisserie forks.

9. If desired, place aluminum foil onto the drip pan. (It makes for easier clean-up!)

10. Select the Roast function and preheat Maxx to 380 degrees Fahrenheit (193 degrees Celsius). Press Rotate button and set Time to 40 minutes.

11. Once the unit has preheated, place the chicken with the rotisserie spit into the oven.

12. When cooking is complete, remove the chicken using the rotisserie handle and,

using hot pads or gloves, carefully remove the chicken from the spit.

13.   Let sit for 10 minutes before slicing and serving.

Nutrition: Calories 311 Fat 11g Carbohydrate 22g Protein 31g

Lemony Rotisserie Lamb Leg

Preparation Time:25 minutes

Cooking Time: 1 hour 30 minutes

Servings: 4

Ingredients:

- pounds (1.4 kg) leg of lamb, boned in
- Marinade:
- tablespoon lemon zest (about 1 lemon)
- tablespoons lemon juice (about 11/2 lemons) - 3 cloves garlic, minced
- 1 teaspoon onion powder - 1 teaspoon fresh thyme
- ¼ cup fresh oregano - ¼ cup olive oil
- 1 teaspoon ground black pepper
- Herb Dressing:
- 1 tablespoon lemon juice (about 1/2 lemon) - ¼ cup chopped fresh oregano
- 1 teaspoon fresh thyme - 1 tablespoon olive oil
- 1 teaspoon sea salt - Ground black pepper, to taste

Directions:

1. Place lamb leg into a large resealable plastic
   bag. Combine the Ingredients: for the
   marinade in a small bowl. Stir to mix well.
   Pour the marinade over the lamb, making
   sure the meat is completely coated. Seal
   the bag and place in the refrigerator.
   Marinate for 4 to 6 hours before air fryer
   grilling. Remove the lamb leg from the
   marinade. Using the rotisserie spit, push
   through the lamb leg and attach the
   rotisserie forks.
2. If desired, place aluminum foil onto the drip
   pan. (It makes for easier clean-up!)
3. Place the lamb leg with rotisserie spit into
   the air fryer grill.
4. Select Toast, set temperature to 350
   degrees Fahrenheit (180 degrees Celsius),
   Rotate, and set Time to 1 hour 30 minutes.
   Baste with marinade for every 30 minutes.
   Meanwhile, combine the Ingredients: for
   the herb dressing in a bowl. Stir to mix
   well.
5. When cooking is complete, remove the
   lamb leg using the rotisserie lift. Using hot

pads or gloves, carefully remove the lamb leg from the spit.

6. Cover lightly with aluminum foil for 8 to 10 minutes.

7. Carve the leg and arrange on a platter, drizzle with herb dressing. Serve immediately.

Nutrition: Calories 306.6 Total Fat 13.5g Saturated Fat 4.8g Total Carbohydrate 6.6g Dietary Fiber 0.3g Sugars 0.5g Protein 37.6g

Chicken Breast with Veggies

Preparation Time:20 minutes

Cooking Time: 30 minutes

Servings: 4

Ingredients:

- deboned chicken breasts
- tbsp. dried Italian herb
- Salt and pepper
- 1 tbsp. paprika
- 1 large carrot, chopped
- 1 large potato, chopped

Directions:

1. Preheat the Power Xl Air Fryer Grill to 150 degrees Celsius or 300 degrees Fahrenheit.
2. Mix all the seasonings and coat the chicken and veggies.
3. Roast the chicken and veggies for 30 minutes.

Nutrition: Calories 140 Fat 0.5g Protein 22g

Simple Air-Fried Beef Roast

Preparation Time:5 minutes

Cooking Time: 38 minutes

Servings: 4

Ingredients:

- 2.5-pound (1.1 kg) beef roast - 1 tablespoon olive oil
- tablespoon Poultry seasoning

Directions:

1. Tie the beef roast and rub the olive oil all over the roast. Sprinkle with the seasoning.
2. Using the rotisserie spit, push through the beef roast and attach the rotisserie forks.
3. If desired, place aluminum foil onto the drip pan. (It makes for easier clean-up!)
4. Place the chicken with rotisserie spit into the air fryer grill.
5. Select Air Fry. Set temperature to 360 degrees Fahrenheit (182 degrees Celsius), and set Time to 38 minutes for medium rare beef.

6. When cooking is complete, remove the beef roast using the rotisserie lift. Using hot pads or gloves, carefully remove the beef roast from the spit.

7. Let cool for 5 minutes before serving.

Nutrition: Calories 358.0 Total Fat 15.5g Saturated Fat 4.5g Total Carbohydrate 0.0g Dietary Fiber 0.0g Sugars 0.0g Protein 50.0g

Air-Fried Lemony-Garlicky Chicken

Preparation Time:10 minutes

Cooking Time: 45 minutes

Servings: 4

Ingredients:

- pounds (1.4 kg) tied whole chicken
- cloves garlic, halved
- whole lemon, quartered
- sprigs fresh rosemary whole
- tablespoons olive oil
- Chicken Rub:
- 1/2 teaspoon fresh ground pepper
- 1/2 teaspoon salt
- 1 teaspoon garlic powder
- 1 teaspoon dried oregano
- 1 teaspoon paprika
- 1 sprig rosemary (leaves only)

Directions:

1. Mix the rub ingredients in a small bowl. Set aside.
2. Place the chicken on a clean cutting board. Ensure the cavity of the chicken is clean.

Stuff the chicken cavity with the garlic, lemon, and rosemary.

3. Tie your chicken with twine if needed. Pat the chicken dry.
4. Drizzle the olive oil all over and coat the entire chicken with a brush.
5. Shake the rub on the chicken and rub in until the chicken is covered.
6. Using the rotisserie spit, push through the chicken and attach the rotisserie forks.
7. If desired, place aluminum foil onto the drip pan. (It makes for easier clean-up!)
8. Place the chicken with the rotisserie spit into the air fryer grill.
9. Select Air Fry, set the temperature to 375 degrees Fahrenheit (190 degrees Celsius). Set the Time to 40 minutes. Check the temp in 5-minute increments after the 40 minutes.
10. At 40 minutes, check the temperature every 5 minutes until the chicken reaches 165 degrees Fahrenheit (74 degrees Celsius) in the breast, or 165 degrees

Fahrenheit (85 degrees Celsius) in the thigh.

11. Once cooking is complete, remove the chicken using the rotisserie lift. Using hot pads or gloves, carefully remove the chicken from the spit.

12. Let the chicken sit, covered, for 5 to 10 minutes.

13. Slice and serve.

Nutrition: Calories 311 Fat 11g Carbohydrate 22g Protein 31g

Roasted Duck

Preparation Time:10 minutes

Cooking Time: 3 hours

Servings: 12

Ingredients:

- lb. whole Pekin duck
- Salt
- garlic cloves chopped
- lemon, chopped
- Glaze
- 1/2 cup balsamic vinegar
- 1 lemon, juiced
- 1/4 cup honey

Directions:

1. Place the Pekin duck in a baking tray and add garlic, lemon, and salt on top.
2. Whisk honey, vinegar, and honey in a bowl.
3. Brush this glaze over the duck liberally.
4. Marinate overnight in the refrigerator.
5. Remove the duck from the marinade and fix it on the rotisserie rod in the
6. Air fryer oven

7. Turn the dial to select the "Air Roast" mode.

8. Hit the Time button and again use the dial to set the cooking Time to 3 hours.

9. Now push the Temp button and rotate the dial to set the temperature at 350 degrees F.

10. Close its lid and allow the duck to roast.

11. Serve warm.

Nutrition: Calories 387 Fat 6g Carbohydrate 37.4g Protein 14.6g

Buttermilk Marinated Chicken

Preparation Time:10 minutes

Cooking Time: 25 minutes

Servings: 6

Ingredients:

- 3-lb. whole chicken
- tablespoon salt
- 1-pint buttermilk

Directions:

1. Place the whole chicken in a large bowl and Drizzle with salt on top.
2. Pour the buttermilk over It and leave the chicken soaked overnight.
3. Cover the chicken bowl and refrigerate overnight.
4. Remove the chicken from the marinade and fix it on the rotisserie rod in the Air fryer oven.
5. Turn the dial to select the "Air Roast" mode.
6. Hit the Time button and again use the dial to set the cooking Time to 25 minutes

7. Now push the Temp button and rotate the dial to set the temperature at 370 degrees F.

8. Close its lid and allow the chicken to roast.

9. Serve warm.

Nutrition: Calories 284 Fat 7.9g Carbohydrate 46g Protein 17.9g

Lamb Kebabs

Preparation Time:5 minutes

Cooking Time: 10 minutes

Servings: 3

Ingredients:

- tablespoon extra-virgin olive oil
- teaspoons cumin powder
- 1 lb. lamb fillet, cut into 1-Inch pieces
- Salt and fresh ground pepper to taste

Directions:

1. Combine all the ingredients in a bowl.
2. Put 2 pieces of lamb onto 6-inch skewers.
3. Choose the air fry option.
4. Cook for 8 minutes at 400 degrees Fahrenheit.
5. Flip halfway through the cooking Time.

Nutrition: Calories 306.6 Total Fat 13.5g Saturated Fat 4.8g Total Carbohydrate 6.6g Dietary Fiber 0.3g Sugars 0.5g Protein 37.6g

Moorish Goat Skewers

Preparation Time:5 minutes

Cooking Time: 6 hours 30 minutes

Servings: 4

Ingredients:

- teaspoon turmeric
- oz. olive oil
- garlic cloves, finely minced
- teaspoon nutmeg, ground
- 1/2 teaspoon, plus 1/2 teaspoon cayenne pepper
- 1 bunch curly parsley, chopped
- oz. fine, plus 2 oz. sherry
- tablespoons cumin seeds, ground
- 1 tablespoon, plus 1 teaspoon sweet Spanish paprika
- 1/2 lemon, squeezed
- lb. goat meat, cut into 1-inch cubes
- Salt to taste

Directions:

1. In a large bowl, mix cumin, nutmeg, turmeric, garlic, parsley, ½ teaspoon

cayenne powder, 1 tablespoon paprika, 7 oz. fine, and olive oil.

2. Add goat meat.

3. Cover and chill for 6 hours or overnight.

4. Thread goat cubes into metal skewers.

5. To create basting liquid, mix 2 oz. sherry, 1/2 teaspoon cayenne pepper, 1 teaspoon paprika, and lemon juice.

6. Choose the grill or use the rotisserie function in your air fryer oven.

7. Set the temperature to 200 degrees Fahrenheit and cook for 15 minutes.

8. Brush basting liquid occasionally.

Nutrition: Calories 274.1 Total Fat 15.7g Saturated Fat 3.5g Total Carbohydrate 10.3g Dietary Fiber 1.1g Sugars 9.0g Protein 21.4g

Roasted Whole Chicken

Preparation Time:5 minutes

Cooking Time: 1 hour and 10 minutes

Servings: 5

Ingredients:

- whole chicken, cleaned
- Rub
- tablespoons oil
- 1 teaspoon onion powder
- 1 teaspoons thyme
- teaspoons paprika
- 1/2 teaspoon cayenne pepper
- 1/2 teaspoon garlic powder
- 1/4 cup fresh thyme, chopped
- 1/4 cup fresh rosemary, chopped
- Salt and pepper to taste

Directions:

1. Combine the rub ingredients in a bowl.
2. Rub the spice mixture all over the chicken.
3. Attach the chicken in the rotisserie spit inside the air fryer oven.
4. Set it to rotisserie.

5. Cook at 350 degrees Fahrenheit for 2 hours.

Nutrition: Calories 127 Fat 0.5g Protein 26g

Spiced Pork Shoulder

Preparation Time:15 minutes

Cooking Time: 55 minutes

Servings: 6

Ingredients:

- teaspoon ground cumin
- 1 teaspoon cayenne pepper
- 1 teaspoon garlic powder
- Salt and ground black pepper, as required
- pounds skin-on pork shoulder

Directions:

1. In a small bowl, mix together the spices, salt and black pepper.
2. Arrange the pork shoulder onto a cutting board, skin-side down.
3. Season the inner side of pork shoulder with salt and black pepper.
4. With kitchen twines, tie the pork shoulder into a long round cylinder shape.
5. Season the outer side of pork shoulder with spice mixture.

6. Insert the rotisserie rod through the pork shoulder.

7. Insert the rotisserie forks, one on each side of the rod to secure the pork shoulder.

8. Arrange the drip pan in the bottom of Kalorik Maxx Air Fryer Oven cooking chamber.

9. Select "Roast" and then adjust the temperature to 350 degrees Fahrenheit.

10. Set the Timer for 55 minutes and press the "Start".

11. When the display shows "Add Food" press the red lever down and load the left side of the rod into the oven.

12. Now, slide the rod's left side into the groove along the metal bar so it doesn't move.

13. Then, close the door and touch "Rotate".

14. When cooking Time is complete, press the red lever to release the rod.

15. Remove the pork from oven and place onto a platter for about 10 minutes before slicing.

16.   With a sharp knife, cut the pork shoulder into desired sized slices and serve.

Nutrition: Calories 445 Total Fat 32.5g Saturated Fat 11.9g Cholesterol 136mg Sodium 131mg Total Carbohydrates 0.7g Fiber 0.2g Sugar 0.2g Protein 35.4g

Seasoned Pork Tenderloin

Preparation Time:10 minutes

Cooking Time: 45 minutes

Servings: 5

Ingredients:

1. 1½ pounds pork tenderloin
2. 2-3 tablespoons BBQ pork seasoning
3. Directions:
4. Rub the pork with seasoning generously.
5. Insert the rotisserie rod through the pork tenderloin.
6. Insert the rotisserie forks, one on each side of the rod to secure the pork tenderloin.
7. Arrange the drip pan in the bottom of Kalorik Maxx Air Fryer Oven cooking chamber.
8. Select "Roast" and then adjust the temperature to 360 degrees Fahrenheit.
9. Set the Timer for 45 minutes and press the "Start".

10. When the display shows "Add Food" press the red lever down and load the left side of the rod into the oven.

11. Now, slide the rod's left side into the groove along the metal bar so it doesn't move.

12. Then, close the door and touch "Rotate".

13. When cooking Time is complete, press the red lever to release the rod.

14. Remove the pork from oven and place onto a platter for about 10 minutes before slicing.

15. With a sharp knife, cut the roast into desired sized slices and serve.

Nutrition: Calories 195 Total Fat 4.8g Saturated Fat 1.6g Cholesterol 99mg Sodium 116mg Total Carbohydrates 0g Fiber 0g Sugar 0g Protein 35.6g

Glazed Pork Tenderloin

Preparation Time:15 minutes

Cooking Time: 20 minutes

Servings: 3

Ingredients:

- 1-pound pork tenderloin
- tablespoons Sriracha
- tablespoons honey
- Salt, as required

Directions:

1. Insert the rotisserie rod through the pork tenderloin.
2. Insert the rotisserie forks, one on each side of the rod to secure the pork tenderloin.
3. In a small bowl, add the Sriracha, honey and salt and mix well.
4. Brush the pork tenderloin with honey mixture evenly.
5. Arrange the drip pan in the bottom of Kalorik Maxx Air Fryer Oven cooking chamber.
6. Select "Air Fry" and then adjust the temperature to 350 degrees Fahrenheit.

7. Set the Timer for 20 minutes and press the "Start".

8. When the display shows "Add Food" press the red lever down and load the left side of the rod into the oven.

9. Now, slide the rod's left side into the groove along the metal bar so it doesn't move.

10. Then, close the door and touch "Rotate".

11. When cooking Time is complete, press the red lever to release the rod.

12. Remove the pork from oven and place onto a platter for about 10 minutes before slicing.

13. With a sharp knife, cut the roast into desired sized slices and serve.

Nutrition: Calories 269 Total Fat 5.3g Saturated Fat 1.8g Cholesterol 110mg Sodium 207mg Total Carbohydrates 13.5g Fiber 0g Sugar 11.6g Protein 39.7g

Crusted Rack of Lamb

Preparation Time: 15 minutes

Cooking Time: 19 minutes

Servings: 4

Ingredients:

- rack of lamb, trimmed all fat and frenched
- Salt and ground black pepper, as required
- 1/3 cup pistachios, chopped finely
- tablespoons panko breadcrumbs
- teaspoons fresh thyme, chopped finely
- 1 teaspoon fresh rosemary, chopped finely
- 1 tablespoon butter, melted
- 1 tablespoon Dijon mustard

Directions:

1. Insert the rotisserie rod through the rack on the meaty side of the ribs, right next to the bone.
2. Insert the rotisserie forks, one on each side of the rod to secure the rack.
3. Season the rack with salt and black pepper evenly.

4. Arrange the drip pan in the bottom of Kalorik Maxx Air Fryer Oven cooking chamber.

5. Select "Air Fry" and then adjust the temperature to 380 degrees Fahrenheit.

6. Set the Timer for 12 minutes and press the "Start".

7. When the display shows "Add Food" press the red lever down and load the left side of the rod into the oven.

8. Now, slide the rod's left side into the groove along the metal bar so it doesn't move.

9. Then, close the door and touch "Rotate".

10. Meanwhile, in a small bowl, mix together the remaining ingredients except the mustard.

11. When cooking Time is complete, press the red lever to release the rod.

12. Remove the rack from oven and brush the meaty side with the mustard.

13. Then, coat the pistachio mixture on all sides of the rack and press firmly.

14. Now, place the rack of lamb onto the cooking tray, meat side up.

15. Select "Air Fry" and adjust the temperature to 380 degrees Fahrenheit.

16. Set the Timer for 7 minutes and press the "Start".

17. When the display shows "Add Food" insert the cooking tray in the center position.

18. When the display shows "Turn Food" do nothing.

19. When cooking Time is complete, remove the tray from oven and place the rack onto a cutting board for at least 10 minutes.

20. Cut the rack into individual chops and serve.

Nutrition: Calories 824 Total Fat 39.3g Saturated Fat 14.2g Cholesterol 233mg Sodium 373mg Total Carbohydrates 10.3g Fiber 1.2g Sugar 0.2g Protein 72g

Beer Can Chicken

Preparation Time:10 minutes

Cooking Time: 40 minutes

Servings: 4

Ingredients:

- Brine

- 2 cups water

- 2 cans beer

- ¼ cup kosher salt

- ½ cup brown sugar

- 8 thyme sprigs

- 3-lb whole chicken, cleaned

- Rub

- 2 tsp. paprika

- tbsp. thyme, dried

- ½ tsp. salt

- ¼ tsp. onion powder

- ¼ tsp. garlic powder

- ¼ tsp. freshly ground black pepper

- tbsp. extra virgin olive oil

Directions:

1. Bring 1 cup water to a simmer in a pot.

2. Dissolve the kosher salt, sugar, and thyme in the simmering water. Add 1 cup water and the beer to the brine.

3. Marinate the chicken in the brine overnight.

4. Combine the rub ingredients in a bowl.

5. Remove the chicken from the brine and pat the chicken dry.

6. Brush the chicken with the olive oil and apply the rub to the chicken.

7. Assemble the Adjustable Skewer Racks with the Rotisserie Shaft and secure the Shaft with the Rotisserie Forks and Set Screws.

8. Set the Shaft through the chicken and tie butcher's twine around

9. the chicken's legs, center, and wings.

10. Set the Shaft into the Kalorik Maxx Air Fryer Oven's Rotisserie Shaft sockets.

11. Press the Power Button and then the Rotisserie Button (400 degrees Fahrenheit for 30 minutes).

12. Carefully remove the chicken using the Fetch Tool.

Nutrition: Calories 311 Fat 11g Carbohydrate 22g Protein 31g

Balsamic-Glazed Chicken Breasts

Preparation Time: 10 minutes

Cooking Time: 19 minutes

Servings: 6

Ingredients:

- Balsamic Glaze
- 2/3 cup balsamic vinegar
- cloves garlic, grated
- ¼ cup Dijon mustard
- ¼ cup honey
- tsp. salt
- ½ tsp. freshly ground black pepper
- 1 cup extra virgin olive oil
- small boneless and skinless chicken breasts

Directions:

1. Whisk the balsamic vinegar, garlic, Dijon mustard, honey, salt, and pepper together in a bowl. Drizzle the olive oil into the glaze while whisking to emulsify the glaze.

2. Marinate the chicken breasts in the marinade for 45 minutes in the refrigerator.

Toss the chicken breasts halfway through the cooking Time (22 ½ minutes).

3. Fold the chicken in half on the Rotisserie Shaft and secure the Shaft with the Rotisserie Forks and Set Screws. Set the Shaft into the Power Air Fryer Oven's Rotisserie Shaft sockets.

4. Press the Power Button and then the Rotisserie Button (400 degrees Fahrenheit for 30 minutes). Brush the chicken with the glaze every 10 minutes while the chicken is cooking.

5. Carefully remove the chicken using the Fetch Tool.

Nutrition: Calories 127 Fat 0.5g Protein 26g

Buttered Broccoli

Preparation Time:5 minutes

Cooking Time: 15 minutes

Servings: 4

Ingredients:

- lb. Broccoli florets – 1 lb.
- tbsp. Butter, melted
- ½ tsp. Red pepper flakes, crushed

- Salt and ground black pepper, as required
- Directions:
- Gather all of the ingredients in a bowl and toss to coat well.
- Place the broccoli florets in the rotisserie basket and attach the lid.
- Arrange the drip pan in the bottom of the Air Fryer Oven cooking chamber.
- Take to the preheated air fryer at 400 degrees Fahrenheit for 15 minutes.
- Serve immediately.

Nutrition: Calories 55 Carbohydrates 6.1g Fat 3g Protein 2.3g

Seasoned Carrots with Green Beans

Preparation Time:5 minutes

Cooking Time: 10 minutes

Servings: 4

Ingredients:

- ½ lb. Green beans, trimmed
- ½ lb. Carrots, peeled and cut into sticks
- tbsp. Olive oil
- Salt and ground black pepper, as required

Directions:

1. Gather all the Ingredients into a bowl and toss to coat well.
2. Place the vegetables in the rotisserie basket and attach the lid.
3. Arrange the drip pan in the bottom of the Air Fryer Oven cooking chamber. Take to the preheated air fryer at 400 degrees Fahrenheit for 10 minutes.
4. Serve hot.

Nutrition: Calories 94 Carbohydrates 12.7g Fat 4.8g Protein 2g

Seasoned Veggies

Preparation Time:5 minutes

Cooking Time: 12 minutes

Servings: 4

Ingredients:

- cup Baby carrots
- 1 cup Broccoli florets
- 1 cup Cauliflower florets
- 1 tbsp. Olive oil
- 1 tbsp. Italian seasoning
- Salt and ground black pepper, as required

Directions:

1. Gather all of the Ingredients into a bowl and toss to coat well.
2. Place the vegetables in the rotisserie basket and attach the lid.
3. Arrange the drip pan in the bottom of the Air Fryer Oven cooking chamber.
4. Take to the preheated air fryer at 380 degrees Fahrenheit for 18 minutes.
5. Serve

Nutrition: Calories 66 Carbohydrates 5.7g Fat 4.7g Protein 1.4g

Paprika Rotisserie-Style Chicken

Preparation Time: 5 minutes

Cooking Time: 80 minutes + marinating Time

Servings: 4

Ingredients:

- (3 ½- 4 lb.) whole chicken
- tbsp salt
- cups buttermilk
- tsp lime juice
- tbsp butter, melted
- 1 tbsp paprika
- Black pepper and sea salt to taste

Directions:

1. Mix the salt, lemon juice, and buttermilk and mix until the salt is dissolved in a large bowl. Submerge the chicken. Cover the bowl and place it in your refrigerator for 2 hours or overnight.

2. Remove the chicken from the fridge, discard the marinade, and pat it dry with kitchen towels. Tie the legs with a butcher's twine and brush with butter. Rub the top

and sides of the chicken with paprika, sea salt, and black pepper.

3. Insert the rotisserie rod through the chicken and attach the forks to secure the rod. Select Roast function on your Kalorik Maxx Air Fryer oven and adjust the temperature to 380 degrees Fahrenheit and the Time to 50 minutes. Slide the chicken into the oven. Press Start/Pause. Make sure the chicken rotates as it cooks.

4. Approximately 10-15 minutes before the end of the suggested cooking Time, start checking for doneness using a meat thermometer. Chicken should have an internal temperature of 165 degrees Fahrenheit. When the chicken is cooked through, remove from the air fryer oven with the removal tool.

5. Put the chicken on a cutting board, and using gloves, carefully remove the chicken from the rod. Cover with foil and leave to rest 10-15 minutes before carving. Serve warm.

Nutrition: Calories 127 Fat 0.5g Protein 26g

Harissa Chicken with Yogurt Sauce

Preparation Time:5 minutes

Cooking Time: 80 minutes + marinating Time

Servings: 4

Ingredients:

- 2 cups sour cream
- Salt and black pepper to taste
- 3 tbsp olive oil
- 3 cloves garlic, minced
- 2 tsp harissa seasoning
- tsp dried dill
- tsp dried tarragon
- 1 (4-lb) whole chicken
- Yogurt Sauce:
- tbsp olive oil
- Salt to taste
- ¼ tsp red pepper flakes, crushed
- 1 cup full-fat yogurt
- 1 tsp dried dill weed

Directions:

1. Mix all the sauce ingredients and place in the refrigerator until ready to use.

2. Put the chicken in a large bowl and pour the sour cream over. Cover with a lid and place in the fridge for 2-3 hours. Pull the chicken from the refrigerator and let it sit for 30 minutes at room temperature.

3. Remove the chicken from the marinade. Tie the legs with a butcher's twine.

4. In a small bowl, whisk the olive oil, garlic, paprika, sage, thyme, tarragon, salt, and pepper to taste. Rub the top and sides of the chicken with the mixture.

5. Insert the rotisserie rod through the chicken and attach the forks to secure the rod.

6. Select Roast function on your Kalorik Maxx Air Fryer oven and adjust the temperature to 380 degrees Fahrenheit and the cooking Time to 60 minutes.

7. Place the chicken in the air fryer oven. Press Start/Pause to begin cooking.

8. When cooking is complete, remove the pan from the oven. Cover with foil and leave to rest 10-15 minutes before carving. Serve the chicken with chilled yogurt sauce.

Nutrition: Calories 274 Fat 12g Fiber 3g Protein 14g Carbohydrates 5g

Spicy Roasted Chicken

Preparation Time:5 minutes

Cooking Time: 75 minutes + marinating Time

Servings: 4

Ingredients:

- (4 lb.) whole chicken
- 4 tbsp olive oil
- tbsp ground coriander
- tsp garlic powder
- tsp onion powder
- tsp chili pepper
- tbsp allspice

Directions:

1. Mix the olive oil, coriander, garlic powder, onion powder, chili pepper, and allspice in a large Ziplock bag; shake to combine well.
2. Place the chicken in the bag and massage to coat. Transfer to the refrigerator and allow marinating for 30 minutes.
3. Select Air Fry function on Air Fryer and adjust the temperature to 380 degrees Fahrenheit. Press Start/Pause to begin cooking.

4. Remove the chicken from the bag, place it on the rotisserie rod, and insert it in the air fryer oven. Roast for 40-50 minutes or until the chicken skin is golden and charred, making sure the chicken rotates as it cooks. Check for doneness with a meat thermometer.

5. Remove and let the chicken sit for 10 minutes before serving.

Nutrition: Calories 127 Fat 0.5g Protein 26g

Greek Rotisserie Lamb Leg

Preparation Time:25 minutes

Cooking Time: 1 hour 30 minutes

Servings: 4 to 6

Ingredients:

- 3 pounds (1.4 kg) leg of lamb, boned in
- For the Marinade:
- tablespoon lemon zest (about 1 lemon)
- tablespoons lemon juice (about 1½ lemons)
- cloves garlic, minced
- 1 teaspoon onion powder
- 1 teaspoon fresh thyme
- ¼ cup fresh oregano
- ¼ cup olive oil
- 1 teaspoon ground black pepper
- For the Herb Dressing:
- 1 tablespoon lemon juice (about ½ lemon)
- ¼ cup chopped fresh oregano
- 1 teaspoon fresh thyme
- 1 tablespoon olive oil
- 1 teaspoon sea salt
- Ground black pepper, to taste

Directions:

1. Place lamb leg into a large resealable plastic bag. Combine the Ingredients: for the marinade in a small bowl. Stir to mix well.

2. Pour the marinade over the lamb, making sure the meat is completely coated. Seal the bag and place in the refrigerator. Marinate for 4 to 6 hours before grilling.

3. Remove the lamb leg from the marinade. Using the rotisserie shaft, push through the lamb leg and attach the rotisserie forks.

4. If desired, place aluminum foil onto the drip pan. (It makes for easier clean-up!)

5. Set the oven to Roast, set temperature to 350 degrees Fahrenheit (180 degrees Celsius), Rotate, and set Time to 1 hour 30 minutes. Press Start to begin preheating.

6. Once preheated, place the lamb leg with rotisserie shaft into the oven. Baste with marinade for every 30 minutes.

7. Meanwhile, combine the Ingredients: for the herb dressing in a bowl. Stir to mix well.

8. When cooking is complete, remove the lamb leg using the rotisserie handle and, using hot pads or gloves, carefully remove the lamb leg from the shaft.

9. Cover lightly with aluminum foil for 8 to 10 minutes.

10. Carve the leg and arrange on a platter, Drizzle with herb dressing. Serve immediately.

Nutrition: Calories 824 Total Fat 39.3g Saturated Fat 14.2g Cholesterol 233mg Sodium 373mg Total Carbohydrates 10.3g Fiber 1.2g Sugar 0.2g Protein 72g

Spicy Rotisserie Chicken

Preparation Time:10 minutes

Cooking Time: 45 minutes

Servings: 4

Ingredients:

- 3 pounds (1.4 kg) tied whole chicken
- 3 cloves garlic, halved
- whole lemon, quartered
- sprigs fresh rosemary whole
- tablespoons olive oil
- Chicken Rub:
- ½ teaspoon fresh ground pepper
- ½ teaspoon salt
- 1 teaspoon garlic powder
- 1 teaspoon dried oregano
- 1 teaspoon paprika
- 1 sprig rosemary (leaves only)

Directions:

1. Mix together the rub ingredients in a small bowl. Set aside.
2. Place the chicken on a clean cutting board. Ensure the cavity of the chicken is clean.

Stuff the chicken cavity with the garlic, lemon, and rosemary.

3. Tie your chicken with twine if needed. Pat the chicken dry.
4. Drizzle the olive oil all over and coat the entire chicken with a brush.
5. Shake the rub on the chicken and rub in until the chicken is covered.
6. Using the rotisserie shaft, push through the chicken and attach the rotisserie forks.
7. If desired, place aluminum foil onto the drip pan. (It makes for easier clean-up!)
8. Select Air Fry, Super Convection of the oven, set the temperature to 375 degrees Fahrenheit (190 degrees Celsius). Set the Time to 40 minutes. Check the temp in 5-minute increments after the 40 minutes. Select Start to begin preheating.
9. Once the unit has preheated, place the chicken with the rotisserie shaft into the oven.
10. At 40 minutes, check the temperature every 5 minutes until the chicken reaches 165 degrees Fahrenheit (74 degrees

Celsius) in the breast, or 165 degrees Fahrenheit (85 degrees Celsius) in the thigh.

11.   Once cooking is complete, remove the chicken using the rotisserie handle and, using hot pads or gloves, carefully remove the chicken from the shaft.

12.   Let the chicken sit, covered, for 5 to 10 minutes.

13.   Slice and serve.

Nutrition: Calories 127 Fat 0.5g Protein 26g

Cornish Hen with Montreal Chicken Seasoning

Preparation Time:5 minutes

Cooking Time: 30 minutes

Servings: 2

Ingredients:

- 2 tablespoons Montreal chicken seasoning
- (1½- to 2-pound / 680- to 907-g) Cornish hen

Directions:

1. Preheat the air fryer to 390 degrees Fahrenheit (199 degrees Celsius).
2. Rub the seasoning over the chicken, coating it thoroughly.
3. Place the chicken in the Rotisserie Spit. Set the Timer and Roast for 15 minutes.
4. Flip the chicken and roast for another 15 minutes.
5. Check that the chicken has reached an internal temperature of 165 degrees Fahrenheit (74 degrees Celsius). Add cooking Time if needed.

Nutrition: Calories 127 Fat 0.5g Protein 26g

Mozzarella and Roasted Tomato Crostini

Preparation Time 30 minutes

Cooking Time:10 minutes

Servings: 6

Ingredients:

- 0.5 cup extra virgin olive oil
- 2 cloves of garlic
- teaspoon dried oregano
- 0.5 teaspoon of sea salt
- 0.5 teaspoon of ground black pepper
- 0.5 crispy baguette, cut into 1/2-inch rounds
- cup of grape tomatoes
- 12 slices of fresh mozzarella
- tablespoons of balsamic glaze
- basil leaves chopped to decorate

Directions:

1. Place the grill plate on the smokeless electric grill and preheat the grill to 350 ° F.

2. Mix the olive oil, and garlic, oregano, salt, and black pepper in a clean bowl to form an olive oil marinade.
3. Rube both sides of all the baguette slice with olive oil marinade.
4. Place the baguette slices on the grill plate and grill on each side until toasted. Remove and reserve.
5. Mix the tomatoes with the rest of the olive oil marinade.
6. Place the tomatoes on the griddle and grill until done.
7. Top each slice of baguette with 1 slice of mozzarella and a tablespoon of tomatoes.
8. Drizzle the balsamic glaze and the rest of the marinade over the crostini.
9. Garnish with basil.

Nutrition: Calories 73 Fat 5 g Carbohydrates 0.9 g Sugar 0.5 g Protein 6.1 g Cholesterol 140 mg

Strips NY with Potatoes

Preparation Time 30 minutes

Cooking Time:10 minutes

Servings: 2

Ingredients:

- small onion, sliced
- Halve 1.5 cup small potatoes
- butter spoons
- sprig of rosemary
- tablespoons of olive oil, divided
- 0.75 teaspoons of sea salt, divided
- 0.75 teaspoons of freshly ground black pepper, divided
- 2 12 ounces NY strip steaks

Directions:

1. Place the grill plate on the smokeless electric grill and preheat the grill to 390 ° F.
2. Put a large piece of aluminum foil and put the onion, potatoes, butter, rosemary, 2 tablespoons. Olive oil, ¼ tsp. Salt and ¼ tsp. black pepper in the foil.

3. Fold the foil and seal it tightly around the ingredients.

4. Rub the steaks with 1 tablespoon. Olive oil, ½ tsp. Salt and ½ tsp. black pepper.

5. The foil-wrapped potatoes should be placed on one half of the grill while on the other half place the steaks. Grill to the desired degree of doneness (roast steaks for approx. 5 minutes per side).

6. When you are done, remove the fillets and let them rest for 5 minutes before serving with the potatoes.

Nutrition: Calories 64 Fat 7 g Carbohydrates 0.8 g Sugar 0.7 g Protein 7.2 g Cholesterol 160 mg

Burgers Filled with Blue Cheese

Preparation time: 15 minutes

Cooking Time:15 minutes

Servings: 4

Ingredients:

- 0.5 teaspoon of sea salt
- 0.5 teaspoon of ground black pepper
- 2 pounds of ground beef
- 3 ounces of cream cheese, softened
- 0.33 cup of blue cheese crumbled
- 3 strips of thickly sliced bacon, cooked and diced
- tablespoon butter, softened
- 4 brioche burger buns
- 0.25 cup margarine

Directions:

1. Place the grill plate on the smokeless electric grill and preheat the grill to 350 degrees.
2. Mix salt, black pepper, and ground beef in a bowl.
3. Divide the ground beef into four balls.

4. Mix and mix the cream cheese, blue cheese, bacon, and butter in a separate bowl.

5. Fill each ground beef ball with some blue cheese mixture, seal the balls and squeeze to form patties.

6. Cook the patties on the grill to the desired degree of doneness. Once that's done, remove and reserve the burgers.

7. Grill butter rolls with margarine and grill rolls (butter side down) until golden brown.

8. Put patties on buns.

Nutrition: Calories 78 Fat 15 g Carbohydrates 1.6 g Sugar 0.9 g Protein 7.2 g Cholesterol 152 mg

Chicken Dinner in Foil

Preparation Time 30 minutes

Cooking Time:40 minutes

Servings: 4

Ingredients:

- 4 boneless and skinless chicken legs
- 8 ounces baby carrots, halved lengthways
- 6 ounces small white potatoes, cut in half
- clove of garlic, chopped
- 1 tablespoon of olive oil
- 1 tablespoon of soy sauce
- 0.25 cup of orange juice
- 0.25 cup sage leaves, chopped

Directions:

1. Place the grill plate on the smokeless electric grill and preheat the grill to 390 degrees.
2. Spread out a large piece of aluminum foil and place all the Ingredients: on the aluminum foil.
3. Fold the foil and seal it tightly around the ingredients.

4. Place foil-wrapped Ingredients: on the grill and cook until the chicken is done.

Nutrition: Calories 73 Fat 5 g Carbohydrates 0.9 g Sugar 0.5 g Protein 6.1 g Cholesterol 140 mg

Breakfast Quesadilla

Preparation Time 15 minutes

Cooking Time:8 minutes

Servings: 1

Ingredients:

- 2 tablespoons of rapeseed oil
- cup of boiled and diced potatoes
- 7 breakfast sausages
- 0.5 small onion, diced
- tablespoons of diced red peppers
- 0.5 teaspoon of paprika
- 0.25 teaspoons of sea salt
- 0.25 teaspoons of ground black pepper
- eggs beaten
- 0.5 cup of grated cheese and cheddar mixture, divided
- 2 8 in. Flour tortillas
- 2 tablespoons of tomato sauce for serving
- 1 sour cream for serving

Directions:

1. Place the grill plate on the smokeless electric grill and preheat the grill to 390 degrees.

2. Pour the rapeseed oil on the grill and grill the potatoes in the oil until golden brown (approx. 8 minutes).

3. At this point, the hot dogs should be added and cook until golden brown.

4. Add onion and paprika and cook for 4 to 5 minutes.

5. Stir in paprika, salt, and black pepper and gradually turn it to mix evenly. Take out and store potatoes.

6. Reduce the grill heat to 320 degrees Fahrenheit and cook the eggs with a ¼ cup cheese mixture.

7. Place 1 tortilla on the grill and cover with eggs, sausage, potatoes, remaining cheese, and the other tortilla.

8. Cook until one side is done, turn the quesadilla over and grill for 2 minutes.

9. Remove the quesadilla, cut into slices, and serve with salsa and sour cream.

Nutrition: Calories: 42kcal, Fat: 0.5g, Carb: 10g, Proteins: 1g

Tuna Steaks with Wasabi Mayonnaise

Preparation Time 30 minutes

Cooking Time:10 minutes

Servings: 2

Ingredients:

- 8 ounces of green beans
- cup baby potatoes, quartered
- 0.5 teaspoon of salt
- teaspoon of ground black pepper, divided
- 0.5 cup plus 3 tbsp. extra virgin olive oil, divided
- 1 tablespoon of soy sauce
- 1 tablespoon of merino
- tablespoons of olive oil
- 12-ounce tuna steaks
- 1 tablespoon wasabi powder
- 0.25 cup of mayonnaise
- 2 tablespoons of Nicosia olives
- 2 cups of mixed green salad
- 2 teaspoons of white balsamic vinegar
- 0.25 teaspoons of chopped fresh tarragon
- 0.75 teaspoons of Dijon mustard, divided

- 0.25 teaspoons of sea salt, divided
- 2 tablespoons of red wine vinegar
- 0.5 clove of garlic, chopped
- 1 pinch of sugar

Directions:

1. Place the grill plate on the smokeless electric grill and preheat the grill to 350 ° F.
2. Combine green beans, potatoes, ½ tsp. Salt, ½ tsp. Put black pepper and ¼ cup extra virgin olive oil in a bowl and stir.
3. Place the green beans and potatoes on the grill and cook them until tender. Remove and reserve the green beans and potatoes and raise the heat of the grill to 450 ° F.
4. Combine soy sauce, merino, and olive oil in a shallow bowl. Put the tuna steaks on the plate and marinate for 10 minutes.
5. Grill the tuna steaks until you have reached the desired degree of cooking (approx. 6 minutes per side). Remove and store fillets.

6. Combine the wasabi powder and mayonnaise in a small bowl to make the wasabi mayonnaise.

7. Combine Nicosia olives, mixed green salad, white balsamic vinegar, tarragon, green beans, potatoes, ½ tsp. Mustard, ¼ tsp. Sea salt, ¼ tsp. black pepper and 3 tbsp. Put the extra virgin olive oil in a second bowl and mix.

8. Combine the red wine vinegar, garlic, sugar, ¼ teaspoon. Mustard, ¼ tsp. Sea salt, ¼ tsp. black pepper and ¼ cup extra virgin olive oil in a third bowl to make the vinaigrette and mix with the salad.

9. Serve the tuna steaks over the Nicosia salad and sprinkle the wasabi mayo with the tuna steaks.

Nutrition: Calories: 52kcal, Fat: 0.7g, Carb: 12g, Proteins:21g

Sweet Potato Pancakes

Preparation time 10 minutes

Cooking Time:10 minutes

Servings: 4

Ingredients:

- 2 tablespoons of rapeseed oil
- 2 eggs
- 2 cups vanilla yogurt
- 2 tablespoons of melted butter
- 0.5 cup of milk
- cup mashed sweet potato
- tablespoons of light brown sugar
- cups of flour
- teaspoons of cinnamon
- 1 teaspoon of baking powder
- 1 teaspoon of baking powder
- 0.5 teaspoons of soda
- 0.5 teaspoon of salt

Directions:

1. Place the grill plate on the smokeless electric grill and preheat the grill to 350 ° F.
2. Heat the rapeseed oil on the grill.

3. Mix the eggs, yogurt, butter, and milk in a bowl.

4. Combine potatoes, brown sugar, flour, cinnamon, baking powder, baking soda, soda, and salt in a separate bowl. Fold the dry Ingredients: under the wet Ingredients: to make a batter.

5. Pour ¼ cup batter onto the skillet and fry the pancakes until golden brown (3-5 minutes per side).

6. Serve the pancakes with maple syrup, sliced bananas, and chopped walnuts.

Nutrition: Calories: 42kcal, Fat: 0.5g, Carb: 10g, Proteins: 1g

Roasted Garlic

Preparation Time:5 Minutes

Cooking Time: 25 Minutes

Servings: 12

Ingredients:

- One medium head garlic
- 2 tsp. avocado oil

Directions:

1. Remove any hanging excess peel from the garlic but leave the cloves covered. Cut off ¼ of the head of garlic, exposing the tips of the cloves
2. Drizzle with avocado oil. Place the garlic head into a small sheet of aluminum foil, completely enclosing it. Place it into the air fryer basket. Adjust the temperature to 400 Degrees F and set the Timer for 20 minutes. If your garlic head is a bit smaller, check it after 15 minutes
3. When completed, garlic should be golden brown and very soft

4. To serve, cloves should pop out and easily be spread or sliced. Store in an airtight vessel in the refrigerator for up to 5 days.

5. You may also freeze individual cloves on a baking sheet, then store together in a freezer-safe storage bag once frozen.

Nutrition: Calories: 11 Protein: 0.2g Fiber: 0.1g Fat: 0.7g Carbs: 1.0g

Roasted Corn

Preparation Time:5 Minutes

Cooking Time: 10 Minutes

Servings: 4

Ingredients:

- Four fresh ears of corn
- Two teaspoons olive oil
- salt and pepper to taste

Directions:

1. Remove the corn husks and wash and pat dry the cob.
2. If you need to, cut down the cob to fit in your basket.
3. Drizzle a little oil over each cob and sprinkle with salt and pepper.
4. Cook at 400 degrees for 10 minutes.

Nutrition: Calories: 100 Sodium: 0 mg Dietary Fiber: 1g Fat: 2.8 g Carbs: 16 g Protein: 2 g

Crunchy Cinnamon Apple Chips

Preparation Time:10 minutes

Cooking Time: 10 minutes

Serves 4

Ingredients:

- 2 apples, cored and cut into thin slices
- 2 heaped teaspoons ground cinnamon
- Cooking spray

Directions:

1. Spritz the air fry basket with cooking spray.
2. In a medium bowl, sprinkle the apple slices with the cinnamon. Toss until evenly coated. Spread the coated apple slices on the pan in a single layer.
3. Place the basket on the air fry position.
4. Select Air Fry, set temperature to 350ºF (180ºC) and set Time to 10 minutes.
5. After 5 minutes, remove the basket from the air fryer grill. Stir the apple slices and return the basket to the air fryer grill to continue cooking.

6. When cooking is complete, the slices should be until crispy Remove the basket from the air fryer grill and let rest for 5 minutes before serving.

Nutrition: Calories: 207cal, Carbs: 17g, Protein: 9g, Fat: 12g.

Spicy Potato Chips

Preparation Time:5 minutes

Cooking Time: 22 minutes

Serves 3

Ingredients:

- 2 medium potatoes, preferably Yukon Gold, scrubbed
- Cooking spray
- 2 teaspoons olive oil
- 1/2teaspoon garlic granules
- 1/4teaspoon paprika
- 1/4 teaspoon plus 1/8teaspoon sea salt
- 1/4teaspoon freshly ground black pepper
- Ketchup or hot sauce, for serving

Directions:

1. Spritz the air fry basket with cooking spray.
2. On a flat work surface, cut the potatoes into ¼-inch-thick slices. Transfer the potato slices to a medium bowl, along with the garlic granules, paprika, olive oil, salt, and pepper and toss to coat well. Transfer the potato slices to the air fry basket.

3. Place the basket on the air fry position.

4. Select Air Fry, set temperature to 392ºF (200ºC), and set Time to 22 minutes. Stir the potato slices twice during the cooking process.

5. When cooking is complete, the potato chips should be tender and nicely browned. Remove from the air fryer grill and serve alongside the ketchup for dipping.

Nutrition: Calories: 217cal, Carbs: 19g, Protein: 8g, Fat: 14g.

Roasted Garlic Dip

Preparation Time:10 minutes

Cooking Time: 20 minutes

Servings: 6

Ingredients:

- head garlic
- ½ tablespoon olive oil
- Directions:
- Slice the top off the garlic.
- Drizzle with the olive oil.
- Add to the air fryer.
- Set it to roast.
- Cook at 390 degrees F for 20 minutes.
- Peel the garlic.
- Transfer to a food processor.
- Pulse until smooth.

Nutrition: Calories: 207cal, Carbs: 17g, Protein: 9g, Fat: 12g.

Crispy Avocado Chips

Preparation Time:15 minutes

Cooking Time: 10 minutes

Serves 4

Ingredients:

- egg
- tablespoon lime juice
- 1/8teaspoon hot sauce
- tablespoons flour
- 3/4cup panko bread crumbs
- 1/4cup cornmeal
- 1/4teaspoon salt
- 1 large avocado, pitted, peeled, and cut into ½-inch slices
- Cooking spray

Directions:

1. Whisk together the egg, hot sauce, and lime juice in a small bowl.
2. On a sheet of wax paper, place the flour. In a separate sheet of wax paper, combine the cornmeal, bread crumbs, and salt.
3. Dredge the avocado slices one at a Time in the flour, then in the egg mixture, finally

roll them in the bread crumb mixture to coat well.

4. Place the breaded avocado slices in the air fry basket and mist them with cooking spray.

5. Place the basket on the air fry position.

6. Select Air Fry, set temperature to 390ºF (199ºC), and set Time to 10 minutes.

7. When cooking is complete, the slices should be nicely browned and crispy. Transfer the avocado slices to a plate and serve.

Nutrition: Calories: 42kcal, Carbs: 3g, Protein: 1g, Fat: 0.5g,

Crispy Carrot Chips

Preparation Time:15 minutes

Cooking Time: 10 minutes

Serves 4

Ingredients:

- 4 to 5 medium carrots, trimmed and thinly sliced
- tablespoon olive oil, plus more for greasing
- 1 teaspoon seasoned salt

Directions:

1. Toss the carrot slices with 1 tablespoon of olive oil and salt in a medium bowl until thoroughly coatcd.
2. Grease the air fry basket with the olive oil. Place the carrot slices in the greased pan.
3. Place the basket on the air fry position.
4. Select Air Fry, set temperature to 390ºF (199ºC), and set Time to 10 minutes. Stir the carrot slices halfway through the cooking Time.
5. When cooking is complete, the chips should be crisp-tender. Remove the basket from

the air fryer grill and allow to cool for 5 minutes before serving.

Nutrition: Calories: 40kcal, Carbs: 5g, Protein: 2g, Fat: 0.7g,

Crispy Apple Chips

Preparation Time:10 minutes

Cooking Time: 10 minutes

Serves 4

Ingredients:

- 4 medium apples (any type will work), cored and thinly sliced
- ¼ teaspoon nutmeg
- ¼ teaspoon cinnamon
- Cooking spray

Directions:

1. Place the apple slices in a large bowl and sprinkle the spices on top. Toss to coat.
2. Put the apple slices in the air fry basket in a single layer and spray them with cooking spray.
3. Place the basket on the air fry position.
4. Select Air Fry, set temperature to 360ºF (182ºC), and set Time to 10 minutes. Stir the apple slices halfway through.
5. When cooking is complete, the apple chips should be crispy. Transfer the apple chips

to a paper towel-lined plate and rest for 5 minutes before serving.

Nutrition: Calories: 42kcal, Carbs: 3g, Protein: 1g, Fat: 0.5g,

Simple Radish Chips

Preparation Time:10 minutes

Cooking Time: 15 minutes

Servings:12

Ingredients:

- 1lb radish, wash and slice into chips
- tbsp olive oil
- 1/4 tsp pepper
- 1tsp salt

Directions:

1. Preheat the air fryer to 375 F.
2. Add all Ingredients into the large bowl and toss well.
3. Add radish slices into the air fryer basket and cook for 15 minutes. Shake basket 2-3 Times while cooking.
4. Serve and enjoy.

Nutrition: Calories 108 Fat 1.4 g Carbohydrates 17.4 g Sugar 2.4 g Protein 7.3 g Cholesterol 0 mg

Cucumber Chips

Preparation Time:10 minutes

Cooking Time: 11 minutes

Servings:12

Ingredients:

- 1lb cucumber
- 1/2tsp garlic powder
- 1tbsp paprika
- 1tsp salt

Directions:

1. Wash cucumber and slice thinly using a mandolin slicer.
2. Preheat the air fryer to 370 F.
3. Add cucumber slices into the air fryer basket and sprinkle with garlic powder, paprika, and salt.
4. Toss well and cook for 11 minutes. Shake halfway through.
5. Serve and enjoy.

Nutrition: Calories 112 Fat 2.4 g Carbohydrates 18.2 g Sugar 2.8 g Protein 5.3 g

Easy Corn and Black Bean Salsa

Preparation Time:10 minutes

Cooking Time: 10 minutes

Serves 4

Ingredients:

- ½ (15-ounce) can corn, drained and rinsed
- ½ (15-ounce) can black beans, drained and rinsed
- ¼ cup chunky salsa
- 2 ounces reduced-fat cream cheese, softened
- ¼ cup shredded reduced-fat Cheddar cheese
- ½ teaspoon paprika
- ½ teaspoon ground cumin
- Salt and freshly ground black pepper, to taste

Directions:

1. Combine the corn, black beans, Cheddar cheese, cream cheese, salsa, cumin, and paprika in a medium bowl. Sprinkle with salt and pepper and stir until well blended.

2. Pour the mixture into a baking dish.

3. Place the baking dish in the air fryer grill.

4. Select Air Fry, set temperature to 325ºF (163ºC), and set Time to 10 minutes.

5. When cooking is complete, the mixture should be heated through. Rest for 5 minutes and serve warm.

Nutrition: Calories 108 Fat 1.4 g Carbohydrates 17.4 g Sugar 2.4 g Protein 7.3 g Cholesterol 0 mg

Cheesy Green Chiles Nachos

Preparation Time:10 minutes

Cooking Time: 10 minutes

Serves 6

Ingredients:

- 8 ounces tortilla chips
- 3 cups shredded Monterey Jack cheese, divided
- 2 (7-ounce) cans chopped green chiles, drained
- (8-ounce) can tomato sauce
- ¼ teaspoon dried oregano
- ¼ teaspoon granulated garlic
- ¼ teaspoon freshly ground black pepper
- Pinch cinnamon
- Pinch cayenne pepper

Directions:

1. Arrange the tortilla chips close together in a single layer on the sheet pan. Sprinkle 1½ cups of the cheese over the chips. Arrange the green chiles over the cheese as evenly

as possible. Top with the remaining 1½ cups of the cheese.

2. Place the pan on the toast position.
3. Select Toast, set temperature to 375ºF (190ºC) and set Time to 10 minutes.
4. After 5 minutes, rotate the pan and continue cooking.
5. Meanwhile, stir together the remaining ingredients in a bowl.
6. When cooking is complete, the cheese will be melted and starting to crisp around the edges of the pan. Remove the pan from the air fryer grill. Drizzle the sauce over the nachos and serve warm.

Nutrition: Calories 98 Fat 1.9 g Carbohydrates 15.4 g Sugar 2.4 g Protein 5.3 g

www.ingramcontent.com/pod-product-compliance
Lightning Source LLC
Chambersburg PA
CBHW061000050726
47592CB00003B/1286